JANUA LINGUARUM

STUDIA MEMORIAE
NICOLAI VAN WIJK DEDICATA

edenda curat

C. H. VAN SCHOONEVELD
Indiana University

Series Minor, 126

HESITATION PHENOMENA IN ADULT APHASIC AND NORMAL SPEECH

by

GERD QUINTING

Georgetown University

1971

MOUTON

THE HAGUE · PARIS

LIBRARY OF CONGRESS CATALOG CARD NUMBER: 75-170008

Printed in Belgium, by NICI, Printers, Ghent.

TABLE OF CONTENTS

LIST OF TABLES

I

THE PROBLEM

A. LINGUISTIC ANALYSIS OF APHASIA

As early as 1935, George K. Zipf (1965) stated the need for linguistic research in deviant speech behavior which he called

> a virgin field of probably tremendous fertility for investigation. It would be interesting to know if and to what extent in pathological English ... normal words are replaced either by neologisms, or by accepted words with abnormally increased or decreased frequencies. A phonemic count of word-salads might be very revealing. Though pathological language represents deviation from the norms while Dynamic Philology is primarily concerned with investigating, yet, as representing deviations, it is of as much value in testing the validity of our investigation, as any deviation from the norm is in any scientific problem. (p. 218)

Bloomfield had mentioned aphasia in the linguistic context very briefly in the second chapter of his monumental book (Bloomfield, 1933). And quite recently an appeal was made by F. Grewel (1963) which calls for the linguist's participation in the study of deteriorated aphasic language.

> Our considerations show that many language disorders must be regarded as cerebral symptoms. Our knowledge of their exact nature, and of their correlation with neurophysiological disorders and with anatomical localization is still very insufficient. Neither their exact phonetic nor their phonemic and linguistic analysis has been studied sufficiently. (p. 84)

In the same year a book appeared by Osgood and Miron (1963) which contains a chapter on linguistics and aphasia plus an outline of Skinner's and Osgood's psycholinguistic models of language behavior regarding their usefulness in theoretical foundations of impaired speech.

An earlier study by Wepman, Bock, Jones and Van Pelt (1956) considered anomia as related to specific reductions in syntactic form classes.

Lenneberg (1960) urges that linguists and psychologists make an effort in examining from their respective disciplines the rich body of physiological data from aphasic patients as published in Penfield and Roberts (1959). This book also includes an important historical chapter on past and present works in the field.

Tikofsky (1966) reports more recent linguistic approaches to the study of aphasia.

The actual amount of work in this field of investigation, nevertheless, has been small. Certainly R. Jakobson's contributions must be mentioned here. His theoretical ideas must still be considered very pertinent and basic to a linguistic approach in the study of language deficit although his conclusions were not founded on much experimental data. The nucleus of his views was expressed already in a monograph (1941) and was subsequently elaborated in more detail in Jakobson (1955, 1956). A further attempt was made by Jakobson (1964) to correlate his linguistic premises to A. R. Luria's aphasia classifications. Tikofsky (1966) points out that

> Jakobson relies heavily on Luria's descriptive classification of aphasia in the development of two other basic dichotomies: limitation versus disintegration and sequence (successivity) versus concurrence (simultaneity). He is able to group Luria's six types so that they will fit into one of his three dichotomies. This permits variation within each dichotomy. Jakobson also finds that the linguistic topology he proposes has an anatomical counterpart in the locus of the lesions which underly the impairments. (p. 271)

Apart from this, the interpretive literature on aphasia, by both linguists and others, is far greater than the literature reporting experimental investigations. Therefore, in this writer's opinion, a major research effort should be the linguist's prime concern since so little descriptive analysis of experimentally gathered data is available. That is to say, it is first and foremost a task of simply describing the speech of brain-injured aphasic patients as thoroughly and in as much detail as feasible.

The taxonomic system of descriptive linguistics as generally applied has to undergo certain changes in order to produce a valid analysis, *e.g.*, on the phonetic level additional symbols for transcription are called for in a linguistic microanalysis of some of the vocal productions as found in cases of jargon aphasia. The descriptive system of linguistics has been developed for the description of NORMAL language and is now confronted with the task of accounting for manifestations of speakers' deviances from the norm. The elaborate apparatus as we know it can be productively applied in the description of impaired verbal behavior of aphasic patients, if minor modifications and adjustments are made. It is also safe to say that for the time being, until a large body of this kind of new data is accounted for, it is premature to venture into attempts at constructing theoretical models (psycholinguistic or otherwise) for deviant verbal behavior, if the goal of these models is ultimately to try to incorporate this data into a general theory of language.

Thus the domain of the linguistic aphasia researcher is at the present time still in an ETIC stage, to borrow Pike's terms, from whence the EMIC stage will develop and make generalized systematic statements about aphasic disorders of speech possible.

In sum, the linguist engaging in speech pathology research should have, at this point, less motivation to theorize and more motivation for developing an adequate descriptive apparatus and technique.

Ultimately these efforts will also contribute to our understanding of normal language functions since the linguist is under obligation to constantly recheck his assumptions about language as new data is added to the already known body of material. For instance, the notion of 'degrees of grammaticalness' as established in generative grammar work could be tested and validated (possibly even refined) in the observed utterances of aphasics. Goodglass and Hunt (1958) have already performed some preliminary research on agrammatism, comparing their results to some of Chomsky's theoretical positions. Two more papers on this phenomenon followed, Goodglass and Berko (1960) and Goodglass (1962).

B. STUDIES IN HESITATION PHENOMENA: AN OVERVIEW OF THE LITERATURE

A review of the relevant scientific literature on hesitation pauses in normal speech, mainly scattered in phonetic and psychological journals, immediately makes it obvious that the amount of work has not been very extensive, *i.e.*, very little quantitative information is available. And to the author's knowledge there has been no SYSTEMATIC and linguistic analysis undertaken dealing with these parameters in aphasic speech.

The reason for the latter situation is that aphasia as a domain of linguistic research is still largely *terra incognita*, a true and exciting frontier of modern linguistics. The bulk of the investigations with a linguistic orientation has focused on problems such as articulation disorders in aphasia, perceptual discrimination of selected speech sounds, and agrammatism.

The first remark made above is directly tied to methodological practices in the formal description of natural languages. Since the linguist's attention is primarily centered on the taxonomic description and functional properties of segmentals and suprasegmental features of the language code, theory construction and subsequent testing, etc., the variables under investigation here have virtually been omitted as they are non-verbal and unfilled pauses are even non-vocal. This accounts for the fact that they are usually declared 'extralinguistic'. Birdwhistell (1965) points to this unjustified delimitation when he writes:

> Silence, except in special cases, is defined as non-communication. Consistent with these premises and according to this logic, communication is defined as a discontinuous single-channel process, fully comprehensible by experiments which test the efficiency of the passage of new information from transmitter to reactive receiver. (p. 6)

The fallacy committed by linguists is this: those physical occurrences in speech that cannot be transcribed are termed 'extralinguistic', thus outside of the realm of linguistics. However, they become properly linguistic when a notational set for description is available. It seems that the linguist in order to analyse language often needs to expand his system of notations, arbitrary as they may be. That is why hesitation forms have been, for the most part, disregarded in analytical procedures in the past. However, there have been other features of speech which once were relegated to non-linguistic status but have since been fully incorporated as significant elements in formal language descriptions, *e.g.*, intonation, as was expressed by Twaddell (1959):

> Those factors of "rasp, overloudness, chuckling," and the like are still usually mentioned as being outside the field of linguistics proper—more or less as intonation was outside the domain some decades ago. However, even those who place the voice qualifiers outside are nowadays, I think, placing them "just outside." Their role in psychiatrically applied linguistic research shows signs of being so crucial that they may before long establish a status as describable elements of a speech system. (p. 151)

Another explanation of why so little attention is paid to these phenomena can be found in the mere nature of the attempts at writing a grammar for *L*. In the transformational-generative framework of syntactic description of sentences, Chomsky (1965) assumes as speaker of these sentences

> an ideal speaker-listener, in a completely homogeneous speech-community, who knows its language perfectly and is unaffected by such grammatically irrelevant conditions as memory limitations, distractions, shifts of attention and interest, and errors (random or characteristic) in applying his knowledge of the language in actual performance ....
>
> ....
>
> [And further] A record of natural speech will show numerous false starts, deviations from rules, changes of plan in mid-course, and so on. (pp. 3-4)

In spite of Chomsky's recognition that the linguistic reality looks different from his premises about the ideal speaker with his intuitive knowledge about all features of his native language which, presumably, all other speakers of that language share with him, it becomes quite clear that hesitation considerations are irrelevant in this particular frame of reference. Pausal phenomena clearly belong to linguistic performance or, in Gleason's (1961) conceptualization, to the expression side of language. (This, of course, is derived from L. Hjelmslev's (1927, 1953) conceptual dichotomy of EXPRESSION PURPORT and CONTENT PURPORT. On the expression plane of language all actually spoken forms are realized.) But Chomsky's goal for linguistic theory is viewed as an attempt at accounting for the speaker's linguistic competence of interpreting and assigning structural descriptions to the infinite set of grammatical sentences that can occur in his native tongue. Thus, for the time being, pausal considerations are not meant to be included in this framework until more data has been accumulated and a more detailed methodology is worked out. Only then will it be possible to relegate them to linguistic performance.

Without doubt, then, hesitation devices are not primary linguistic data per se. That is probably why there is not much point, at least in the present state of linguistics, in incorporating them in structural descriptions of grammar, although these elements are present in real linguistic corpora all the time. Even so, we are more inclined to accept Birdwhistell's (1965) notion of human communication as being a multi-channel system, *i.e.*, considering the TOTAL communicative behavior of speakers there is sufficient validity to include the hesitational phenomena in it. Further evidence why they definitely should NOT be ranked as 'extralinguistic' comes from experimental results of Goldman-Eisler (1964) where it is stated that

> An average of about 40-50 percent of utterance time is occupied by pauses (Goldman-Eisler, 1961c).
> These measurements make it evident that pausing is as much part of the act of speaking as the vocal utterance of words itself and this suggests that pausing may be essential to the generation of spontaneous speech. (pp. 98-99)

Therefore, we have to conceive of hesitation pauses as a very basic feature in linguistic performance. Independent of a speaker's educational, socio-economic, or dialect background, there will always be gaps and breaks in the linguistic stream where he self-interrupts the vocal-verbal output. Of course, they may occur more frequently in some speakers than in others and admittedly in some speakers they may certainly be considered as an idiosyncratic characteristic of speech, part of a person's idiolect, so to speak. But the fact is also undeniable that even in a lecture delivered from a written manuscript the well-formed grammatically non-deviant sentences are hardly ever read off the paper without inserted delays and repetitions in the spoken discourse. Goldman-Eisler (1958a) acknowledges this point by stating:

> Two factors operate in speech making it a discrete rather than a continuous performance. (1) Biological necessity forces even the most fluent speaker to stop at more or less regular intervals in order to get air into the lungs. (2) Beside these physically unavoidable halts imposed on every speaker, fluency in speech is frequently blocked psychologically by hesitations. (p. 64)

Turning to some of the research efforts dealing with hesitation types, one encounters various approaches to this problem. Those with a linguistic focus will be considered first.

Goldman-Eisler (1958b and 1958c), who has been a major contributor in this field, asked subjects to guess experimental sentences from a known preceding context and found that pauses occurred at points of uncertainty of prediction. Another finding indicated that the majority of silent pauses preceded content words. This latter result was confirmed by Maclay and Osgood (1959). These two authors investigated the frequency and syntactic environments of hesitation devices. Among those were filled and unfilled pauses. Goldman-Eisler (1961a) analysed further these variables and proposed a correlation of filled pause to emotional factors and of unfilled pause to cognitive activity. In another paper (1961b) she concluded that subjects paused more for the same amount of speech when they summarized the message contained in cartoons than when they described them. Henderson, Eisler and Skarbek (1966) analysed recorded interviews, establishing a possible unit of relatively long pause periods with short utterances and periods of relatively short pauses and long utterances, refuting, they felt, a simple Markovian model of speech production. Schwartz and Jaffe (1968), although observing also these same alternating patterns, nevertheless interpreted them as an example of a Markov process.

The topic of syntactic environments and hesitation distributions was again pursued by Blankenship and Kay (1964). They corroborate the premise that the location of hesitations falls at points of both lexical and structural uncertainty, as advanced by Goldman-Eisler (1958b). But Tannenbaum *et al.* (1965) contradict the latter in that they report no difference between high and low transition probabilities of words following a hesitation.

A study somewhat outside the previous group by Tannenbaum, Williams and Wood (1967) discussed hesitation types, comparing verbal and written modalities in regard to encoding behavior.

Two other papers which do not directly pertain to linguistic considerations are those by Mahl (1956) and Levin and Silverman (1965). The former investigates two hesitation phenomena in the context of anxiety manifestations as observed in psychotherapy interviews. The latter study aims at relating several variables like filled pause, unfilled pause, number of words, amount of speaking time in seconds to two speaking settings and to personality characteristics in children.

Still another paper by Livant (1963) addresses itself to the behavior of pauses in a mathematical framework.

Miller (1963) reports case histories of all three general aphasic syndromes, expressive, receptive and amnesic. He lists data of Weisenberg and McBride's patients and comments on a case of receptive dysfunction as reported by K. Goldstein. These illustrations were checked for the three types of speech disorders and mention of hesitancy was found in all of them. Jones and Wepman (1965) report frequent pausing in the disorder that they have called semantic aphasia. Of course, these were only observations that aphasic speech sometimes was hesitant. No further investigation or description was undertaken.

This survey, taken as a whole, is an indicator of how little is known and understood about these non-verbal but seemingly necessary features that accompany linguistic events when normals speak, let alone their significance in aphasic disturbances.

Speech occurs in real time as a continuous sequence of physical events. This much is obvious. Yet linguists and psychologists have no way of knowing how the brain processes speech temporally, if so, or in what order speech is structured prior to the actual vocal output, *i.e.*, the exact functioning nature of the encoding/decoding process is virtually unknown. References to internal states of brain activity involving the formulation of speech must therefore be considered more as speculation than as actual evidence. In terms of hesitation phenomena this problem is particularly brought into relief. Although filled pauses are overt, what mental behavior is going on in the organism during a period of silence (unfilled pause)[1] is shrouded by the experimenter's inability to make this information amenable to direct analysis. Birdwhistell (1965) mentioned this problem as it pertains to the analysis of kinesic behavior.

> We know far too little about the other communicative modalities to do more than hypothesize about such relationships between the body motion during silence as related to other modalities as well as that which is demanded for the performance of spoken language. (p. 43)

A great proportion of the literature cited above is unsatisfactory to proper linguistic concerns since the variables dealt with are often linked to an information theoretic model, linear and probabilistic. Yet Chomsky (1957) demonstrated convincingly the inadequacy of this type of model for linguistic description.

The impetus for this investigation was generated by the Maclay/Osgood paper (1959). Four types of hesitation phenomena were treated in this study. These were:

(1) Filled Pauses, those vocalized hesitation phones conventionally represented as [ε, æ, r̩, ə, m̩];
(2) Unfilled Pauses, those periods of non-speech in utterances;
(3) Repeats, superfluous repetitions of words that do not contribute to the semantics of an utterance;

[1] Unfilled pause referred to hereafter as UP.

(4) False Starts, all abortive beginnings of utterances. A distinction between retraced FS and non-retraced FS was made, *i.e.*, the speaker either corrected himself or failed to do so.

Their data consisted of tape-recorded and subsequently transcribed speech material taken from twelve subjects participating in a conference. Using the test frames of Fries (1952), the authors located the hesitation types and accounted for the syntactic environments among which they were distributed. The analysis yielded the following results:

(a) Both filled and unfilled pauses precede lexical words more frequently than function words.[2] However, filled pauses occur more often before function words whereas unfilled pauses occur more often before lexical words.
(b) Filled pauses were found more at phrase boundaries, unfilled pauses more within them.
(c) False starts when retraced involve lexical items, and repeats, function words.

Of these variables only (1) and (2) were examined in this research. For example, it would be very difficult to determine the borderline between repeats and manifestations of perseveration as found in aphasic speech.

Result (a) was considered the basis for this study, involving a population of aphasic patients and a population of normal controls.

The nature of the study is necessarily exploratory since little research based on a systematic analysis of these parameters in aphasic speech has been conducted. In addition, for descriptive purposes a body of quantitative data is necessary in order to give validity to the analysis and generalizations derived from the source material.

Osgood and Maclay proposed a non-random distribution of pausal types. The objective here is to ascertain whether aphasics would likewise exhibit this same patterning.

[2] The authors use LEXICAL for what Fries (1952) called "four major form classes". They follow Fries exactly in regard to function word classes.

Before outlining the basic apparatus used for obtaining the relevant data, a comment on the notion of PAUSE as established in linguistics as opposed to HESITATION, as conceived here, is in order.

Maclay/Osgood (1959) make this distinction well when they state:

> there is one basic difference between pause and hesitation: hesitations, as we define them, refer to events that are relatively gross and easily observable, while the juncture-pauses of linguistic theory are quite short in duration and much harder to observe and record. (p. 20)

That is to say that linguists do recognize and have established so-called juncture phonemes,[3] occurring at boundaries of phonological or syntactic units. These pauses are viewed as being linguistic. The suprasegmental phoneme /+/ is a boundary marker to account for differences in otherwise identical sequences of segmental phonemes. But this interrupted transition at morpheme or word boundary is inaudible in a continuous speech sample. The hesitations discussed here, however, are longer in duration and are not necessarily distributed at syntactic juncture points.

For operational purposes we refer to a filled pause as any of the vocal fillers mentioned above.[4] Although a repetition of the same word could be regarded as a FP[5], such incidences were not counted as such.

The criteria for UP are discussed below.

[3] A great many studies presenting elaborate formulations of juncture in both post-Bloomfieldian and Chomskian frameworks have been assembled. An example of the former would be Moulton's study (1947) and of the latter a key article by Chomsky, Halle and Lukoff (1956).

[4] That these devices existing in English are not universal was pcinted out to the author by O.L. Chavarria-Aguilar. In his dialect of Latin American Spanish, a word, *este*, marks a filled pause (personal communication).

[5] FP stands for filled pause.

II

SUBJECTS, APPARATUS AND METHODOLOGY

A. SUBJECTS

In selecting the aphasic population, three preconditions had to be met in order that a subject qualify for inclusion in the experiment:

(1) That there be evidence of aphasia, *i.e.*, S had incurred injury to brain tissue with subsequent damage to speech and language processes;
(2) That the individual's speech be voluntary, *i.e.*, functional in the sense that verbal output occurs without prompting;
(3) That the patient be a native speaker of English.

It also follows from the above that all participating aphasics were adults who at one time were accomplished fluent speakers, having mastered their native language. One S was an adolescent but was considered a mature speaker of his language.

At the beginning of the research when the pause measurement device was other than the one ultimately used, E began recording aphasics until 14 had been taped. The microphone used was the UHER M-514 (table microphone). Unfortunately, this data had to be discarded when the computer pause analysis (outlined below) was substituted for the methodology of measuring pause durations mechanically by tape loop. Of the original population only two of the 14 tapes could be retained since the level of surface noise on all other tapes was too high. Considering the computer's sensitivity threshold for noise, working with this data would have definitely confounded final results. But after the computer program had been written and tested and retested, it turned out that even the aforementioned two tapes were not qualified for pause length analysis.

Thus an additional 8 Ss were recorded with a much improved technique yielding greater fidelity and above all a much reduced level of extraneous noise. In discussing pausal analysis reference will, therefore, always be made to this second population (N = 8), whereas for the linguistic analysis we consider an N of 10, adding the two Ss mentioned above.

The very first step in finding appropriate Ss was to observe patients in a linguistic situation, either in individual or group therapy sessions at their respective rehabilitative institutions. By sitting in on these sessions, E gained a fairly good impression of the patient's level of volitional speech—S interacting on various verbal tasks with the speech therapist. In addition, E was given the opportunity, after the speech therapist had terminated her work, to elicit a speech sample from one or two pictorial stimuli that were similar to those used in all of our taped sessions. A brief free speech sample was elicited by asking S a few everyday questions. It also gave E a chance to introduce himself to the patient by stating E was conducting a study of aphasic speech.

This personal screening technique to assess a patient's baseline behavior turned out to be quite helpful since it provided an indication of who displayed an aphasic symptomatology that was either too severe or too mild to contribute useful data.

The etiology of the speech deficit was unknown in only one of the cases; in another it was carotid artery surgery; and cerebrovascular accidents accounted for the remaining eight. The period of time between onset of the speech impairment and the recordings ranged from five weeks to thirty-one months. In four Ss it was less than one year; in four others it was between one and two years; in two it was two years or more. Their ages ranged from sixteen to seventy-three (average age: 54.2 years). Seven patients were men, three were women. All of them were enrolled in professional speech therapy programs; some as out-patients and two as bed-to-chair patients in a hospital.

The population as a whole was rather homogeneous with regard to the following parameters:

(1) The majority of Ss displayed a moderate aphasia resulting from vascular lesions. Some, however, were rather severely impaired and the specific clinical diagnoses of the CVAs were different, which was reflected in their different levels of linguistic performance;
(2) All Ss showed sufficient vocal production to yield a workable sample;
(3) All were undergoing speech therapy.

Description of the Ten Aphasic Patients

Aphasic Patient A1[1]

Medical data and diagnosis:[2] a phone designer, aged 54; a polio victim since age 2, he suffered a CVA on August 8, 1967, with right hemiplegia and expressive aphasia.[3]

Statistical data:[4]

Ave[5]	=	2.55	SD	=	4.07
Mode[6]	=	.74	Median	=	1.38
NUM[7]	=	721	SUM[9]	=	1839.56
LongP[8]	=	0	Kshort[10]	=	326

1 Throughout this study *A* represents an aphasic subject. The number following the *A* indicates a particular aphasic. A9 and A10 were the aphasics not included in the computational analysis.
2 All medical information was supplied by referral agencies.
3 Howes (1964) criticized the clinical subcategorization of aphasics like "receptive", "expressive", etc., but despite this criticism, these labels are, nevertheless, helpful since they do somewhat describe the condition.
4 The statistical data presented in this chapter concern only unfilled pauses.
5 Average pause length in seconds, for the elicited speech sample.
6 The preferred pause in seconds, *i.e.*, the one occurring most often.
7 Total number of pauses exceeding threshold value of 260 msec (see below).
8 Number of pauses above upper bound.
9 Total length of pause periods in seconds.
10 Total number of pauses below threshold value.

Aphasic Patient A2

Medical data and diagnosis: a security policeman, aged 56; on August 17, 1967, he suffered a thrombosis of the left middle cerebral artery resulting in hemiplegia of the right extremities, a mild facial paresis and aphasia. He was hospitalized the same day and remained so for four weeks, followed by a four-week stay in a convalescent home. The aphasia was primarily expressive with a mild receptive component. There appeared to be mild dyslexia and also mild motor involvement of the articulators. Recovery and rehabilitation of language skills have been good. There was fluctuation from day to day in expressive ability. There remains nominal aphasia to some degree but it is not severe.

Statistical data:

Ave	=	1.79	SD		2.76
Mode	=	.26	Median	=	1.04
NUM	=	1343	SUM	=	2433.68
LongP	=	1	Kshort	=	1415

Aphasic Patient A3

Medical data and diagnosis: a high school junior, aged 16; he was admitted to the hospital on September 14, 1968, where a total aphasia was diagnosed. There was complete paralysis of the right limbs and spasticity; right visual field defect and right facial weakness; moderate expressive aphasia with a mild to moderate receptive component and mild dysarthria; there seemed to be no clue as to what caused the dysfunction.

Statistical data:

Ave	=	1.02	SD	=	1.30
Mode	=	.34	Median	=	.88
NUM	=	1857	SUM	=	1942.32
LongP	=	1	Kshort	=	1756

Aphasic Patient A4

Medical data and diagnosis: a housewife, aged 68; she developed a right-sided hemiplegia in her leg and arm and aphasia after carotid artery surgery, which was performed on March 13, 1966. She was severely impaired in the area of expressive language which involved an articulatory deficit reflected in fricatives and polysyllabic words; she manifested anomia and many syntactic problems such as omission of conjunctions, pronouns, and prepositions. Her reading ability was limited to single words and her writing behavior was non-functional.

Statistical data:

Ave	=	3.14	SD	=	4.93
Mode	=	.30	Median	=	1.76
NUM	=	646	SUM	=	2006.38
LongP	=	1	Kshort	=	1100

Aphasic Patient A5

Medical data and diagnosis: a supervisor in data processing, aged 41; she incurred aphasia secondary to a cerebral embolus which occurred during open heart surgery, performed on April 5, 1967. The surgery was done to replace the mitral valve. The patient was unconscious for two weeks following surgery. There was also a temporary right-sided paresis which left no residuals.

Statistical data:

Ave	=	2.13	SD	=	3.58
Mode	=	.26	Median	=	1.16
NUM	=	837	SUM	=	1798.34
LongP	=	0	Kshort	=	1721

Aphasic Patient A6

Medical data and diagnosis: a housewife, aged 46; she had cardiac involvement in childhood and suffered a CVA in 1966 due to embolism from subacute bacterial endocarditis; she had right hemiparesis and both visual fields impaired but only at the time of hospitalization.

Statistical data:

Ave	=	1.22	SD	=	1.73
Mode	=	.38	Median	=	.84

NUM	= 949	SUM	= 1203.66
LongP	= 1	Kshort	= 1080

Aphasic Patient A7

Medical data and diagnosis: a retired machinist, aged 73; on March 6, 1966, he suffered a cerebral thrombosis affecting speech and producing right hemanopsia; he recovered almost complete language and speech. On September 3, 1968, he suffered a CVA resulting in paralysis of his right arm and leg and aphasia.

Statistical data:

Ave	= 2.44	SD	= 4.04
Mode	= .26	Median	= 1.24
NUM	= 603	SUM	= 1476.32
LongP	= 1	Kshort	= 1179

Aphasic Patient A8

Medical data and diagnosis: a retired marble and tile setter, aged 72; he suffered a CVA due to thrombosis, branch of left middle cerebral artery (no prior history of CVA); substernal thyroid goiter; diabetes mellitus; arteriosclerotic heart disease with atrial fibrillation; he was well two days prior to admission to the hospital (October 28, 1968), when he suddenly developed partial expressive and receptive aphasia, marked reduction in strength of his right hand and arm. His right leg was without deficit and he had no difficulty ambulating; his major difficulty was perseveration (spontaneously repetitive speech) and remembering words, particularly specific place names. However, his sentence structure was normal.

Statistical data:

Ave	= 3.58	SD	= 5.58
Mode	= .30	Median	= 1.82
NUM	= 718	SUM	= 2531.28
LongP	= 1	Kshort	= 959

Aphasic Patient A9

Medical data and diagnosis: a camera supervisor, male, aged 51; CVA onset occurred in May 1965 with right hemiplegia; the second

CVA occurred in October 1965 and a third CVA in February 1967.

Aphasic Patient A10

Medical data and diagnosis: an employee in patent department of manufacturing firm, male, aged 65; he suffered left-sided CVA on April 15, 1968, with resultant right-sided hemiparesis; heart attack and mild CVA in 1967.

DESCRIPTION OF THE TEN NORMAL CONTROL SUBJECTS

We define NORMALS as individuals who exhibit no evidence of cortical insult to brain tissue, either presently or in their past history. The normals used as matching control Ss were matched on the basis of subject sex, age and educational background. Chronological age was matched within a range of five years.

Normal Control Subject N1[11]

A maintenance and housekeeping supervisor, male, aged 50.

Statistical data:

Ave	=	1.75	SD	=	2.75
Mode	=	.28	Median	=	1.20
NUM	=	742	SUM	=	1324.16
LongP	=	1	Kshort	=	2620

Normal Control Subject N2

An office manager, male, aged 55.

Statistical data:

Ave	=	1.72	SD	=	2.87
Mode	=	.42	Median	=	1.04
NUM	=	237	SUM	=	438.42
LongP	=	1	Kshort	=	1520

[11] Throughout this study *N* represents a normal subject. The number following the *N* indicates a particular normal who is matched to the aphasic with the same number.

Normal Control Subject N3

A high school junior, male, aged 16.

Statistical data:

Ave	= 1.12	SD	= 1.87
Mode	= .36	Median	= .84
NUM	= 333	SUM	= 424.50
LongP	= 1	Kshort	= 836

Normal Control Subject N4

A housewife, aged 63.

Statistical data:

Ave	= 1.05	SD	= 1.81
Mode	= .26	Median	= .70
NUM	= 429	SUM	= 506.30
LongP	= 1	Kshort	= 1731

Normal Control Subject N5

A housewife, aged 40.

Statistical data:

Ave	= .97	SD	= 1.39
Mode	= .32	Median	= .88
NUM	= 535	SUM	= 579.16
LongP	= 0	Kshort	= 2564

Normal Control Subject N6

A substitute clerical worker, female, aged 47.

Statistical data:

Ave	= 1.30	SD	= 1.98
Mode	= .26	Median	= 1.02
NUM	= 442	SUM	= 620.24
LongP	= 1	Kshort	= 1681

Normal Control Subject N7

A mechanical engineer, male, aged 74.

Statistical data:

Ave	= .79	SD	= 1.70

Mode	= .28	Median	= .58
NUM	= 437	SUM	= 408.52
LongP	= 0	Kshort	= 2049

Normal Control Subject N8

A grocery store co-owner, male, aged 69.

Statistical data:

Ave	= 1.05	SD	= 1.84
Mode	= .26	Median	= .72
NUM	= 608	SUM	= 693.06
LongP	= 0	Kshort	= 1876

Normal Control Subject N9

A film technician, male, aged 54.

(Data were used for linguistic analysis only; taped material was not of sufficiently good quality to yield data by computer analysis.)

Normal Control Subject N10

A facilities engineer, aged 60.

(Data used for linguistic analysis only.)

B. APPARATUS

Elicitation Material

There were two interview sessions for each aphasic patient, and one for each normal S. In Task 1 Ss were asked to describe a set of 38 pictorial stimuli. In Task 2, E asked some everyday questions for S to answer thus obtaining a free speech sample. Each aphasic was seen twice on different days to complete both tasks, whereas the normals completed both tasks in one session on the same day.

The description task is basically a continuation of what the aphasic was exposed to in speech therapy, *viz.*, the naming and describing of objects and concrete events from, for example, the *Peabody Language Development Kit* (1965). The entire corpus

elicited in Task 1 can be considered a sustained narrative.
The pictorial material was taken from the following:

The Family of Man (1955)
27 black and white photographs

Sapon's (1957) *Pictorial Linguistic Interview Manual* (PLIM)
6 pen and ink sketches (these are contained in Part III of the Manual)

4 cardboard color pictures (No. 2210, Buffalo: Kenworthy Educational Service)

1 black and white newspaper photograph

With the exception of the color pictures, the stimulus material was mounted on scrapbook paper.

The taping sessions for four aphasics were conducted at the patients' homes; another four were held at a Hearing and Speech Center in acoustically treated soundproof rooms, and two were recorded in a hospital room. Six were tape recorded in the morning, four in the early afternoon. Except for two, all normals were tape recorded in their residences.

The elicitation material is a constant for all Ss in both populations. Before each recording session E used to read the standard instruction for Task 1:

I will show you some pictures and I would like you to look at them carefully and describe what you see. Tell me what is in the picture and what it is about. You have all the time you want for each picture.

Usually E would face S at a table and S would be exposed to one stimulus at a time. As soon as one picture was described, E would place the next one in front of S. The order of presentation was fixed since all pictures were numbered. In this narrative task, S would produce speech without being interrupted. There was no one way of correctly describing the stimuli or no incorrect way either. E never spoke during the entire session in order to avoid the recording of his voice so as not to add extraneous acoustic material. An occasional nod of the head was provided.

This procedure proved to be very convenient to elicit a large sample. We are in agreement with Howes (1964) who found:

Satisfactory 5,000-word samples have been obtained in this way from more than 60 aphasic patients. Patients with extreme paucity of speech naturally cannot supply a sample of this size, and consequently are not represented in our series; yet even patients whom one would suppose to be incapable of producing so many words in spontaneous discourse, when given plenty of time and a congenial interviewer, have been able to produce satisfactory samples. (p. 62)

In selecting elicitation material, it was recognized that there is no neutral stimulus for any subject. There was no concern about HOW a subject perceived and interpreted a stimulus, *i.e.*, this was not a task of character identification, which is a criterion, *e.g.*, for the Thematic Apperception Test (TAT) stimulus cards; but the emphasis was rather on quantity of output. The photographs in *The Family of Man* collection are concrete, action-packed and communicate experiences that are genuinely American or universal. They were enjoyed by most Ss.

To keep the set of questions asked by E somewhat uniform in Task 2, an attempt was made to repeat some of them with each S. However, this could often not be attained, since E in this kind of setting took his cues for the next question from what S had just said. Thus a bona fide conversation was often established.
Some of the questions were:

- What is your favorite TV show and why?
- Could you tell me something about your family?
- Did you ever go on a fishing trip or belong to the Boy Scouts?
- What kind of music do you like best?

The data of Task 2 were not subjected to a computer analysis of pause durations since E's speech was taped also.[12]

To complete Task 1 it took the aphasic patients 45 minutes on the average and the normal controls 20 minutes. Usually 15-20 minutes were spent to elicit a free speech sample.

[12] In a few cases the E's voice was inaudible due to the type of microphone used. Nevertheless, Task 2 was not considered for pause analysis by the computer.

All tapes were transcribed in conventional orthography, attempting to obtain as close a verbatim approximation as possible, *i.e.*, the typescripts were not edited in any way.

In sum, the nature of the elicitation material and the setting of the recording sessions contributed greatly to the elicitation of spontaneous speech. Ss were relaxed enough to speak freely in the environments with which they were most familiar, *viz.*, their home residences or the rehabilitative agencies.

Speech Recording Equipment

All tape recordings were made on Audiotape, Type 651 (600 ft. of 1 1/2 mil Acetate), using the UHER 4000 Report-L model tape recorder. The recording speed for all Ss was constant at 1 7/8 ips. Since this tape recorder accepts only 5-inch reels, a recording made at the above speed yields one hour of taped speech data per track. This speed was chosen to ensure an uninterrupted session, thus avoiding the necessity of turning the tape to the second track.

In order to improve on the problems of extraneous noise pickup during the recording of speech data, E had a KOSS headset modified, *i.e.*, the earphones along with the wiring were removed, thus allowing the Ss to hear when E spoke to them during Task 2. In addition, an adjustable curved boom arm was attached to one of the cups. At its end an AKG microphone, Model D58E, was installed. This is a dynamic noise-cancelling microphone which has been developed for close range voice applications in noisy surroundings. Its impedance is 200 ohms, the frequency range is 70 ... 12,000 cps; it is 1 5/8" long, 13/16" in diameter and weighs 1.1 ozs. The microphone wire, running along the underside of the boom through the rubber-cushioned metal headband, was connected to a SHURE (Model No. A95A) line-matching transformer. The latter was connected to the tape recorder input.

This unit, relatively light-weight, had the advantage that the speech distance from the microphone, of approximately two inches, was constant, no matter in which direction S turned his head. It also made it possible to turn the volume control down during recordings, which was a further protection against noise pickup other than speech. Thus we obtained high-quality voice reproductions.

Before the actual recording session took place, the headset was placed in position to familiarize Ss with the apparatus and to make adjustments relative to their comfort. There was no discernible loss of spontaneity but, nevertheless, wearing a headset and being recorded is not a wholly natural linguistic setting. It is, however, necessary to use this device in order to obtain clean data, although the latter can never really be acquired inasmuch as Ss occasionally cough, clear their throats, interrupt silences by hard breathing or noisy movements. These factors remain present in the data and it is experimentally and technically not feasible to achieve control over these factors even in an unechoic chamber. However, for a computer linguistic noise and non-linguistic extraneous noise are indistinguishable.

C. METHODOLOGY

Computer Program for Measurement of Pause Length

This program locates pauses in utterances of tape recorded speech and measures them automatically. Two computers are involved in the analysis, an EAI (Electronic Associates, Inc.) 680 A/D Converter and an IBM 7700. They were connected to each other.

The tape machine was wired to the A/D Converter, to an oscilloscope and an oscillograph. After the silence threshold and threshold sensitivity had been typed in in volts on a teletypewriter, the tape was started. A visual display on the Converter indicated whether the data was properly converted or not. Lights went on for voice, off for silence.

This program contains an EOB (end-of-block) interrupt routine. It is executed every time an EOB interrupt occurs from the data subchannel. The channel is programmed to interrupt every 20 data points. Since each point is taken at .5 msec intervals, a block of 20 data values, representing voltages in A/D converter code, represents a 10 msec time block. This block is analyzed to determine if the average voltage in this 10 msec interval was above the silence level. Since the tape was run at double speed (3.75 ips), a 10 msec time block represents 20 msec of tape time. Thus 20 msec was the threshold for a silent pause.

The computed data, in the last stage, were received by the IBM 1442 card reader/punch where they were punched on binary data cards, measurements of 26 pause durations per card. This card deck was then fed into an IBM 360 computer in order to obtain a listing of all pause lengths (see appendix).

Computer Program for Pause Length Distribution Analysis

This program, written for the IBM 7700 computer, analyzes the same binary data produced by the previous analysis and finds the frequency distribution of the pause lengths. It also calculates the mean and median scores, the SD and the mode of the data. Each card deck is fed into the 1442 card reader and labeled results are printed out on a Selectric typewriter (see appendix).

In order to compute only those silences that are veritable hesitations and not gaps at juncture boundaries between syllables or aspiration features of voiceless stop consonants, a lower bound of .26 seconds was chosen. Thus Kshort, a fixed integer variable, lists the number of pauses that were below this lower bound. These were rejected for computation. This value was motivated by considerations that Goldman-Eisler (1958b) stated:

> Greater precision of measurement would bring into the range of distinction a different level of speech production, namely the phonetic one. (Pauses up to 0.20 or even 0.25 seconds, though rare, might occur as part of ritardando effects, or articulatory shifts or between plosives.) To be quite certain that these were not included, the gaps in the visual record classified as pauses had to be equivalent to durations of not less than 0.25 seconds. (p. 99)

Brady (1965) investigating the presence of speech and pause periods on a telephone circuit, also established a 200 msec threshold for those pauses that are not articulatorily conditioned.

The upper bound in our computations on pause length distribution was set at 33 seconds since this was the longest pause occurring in any of the speech samples. Pauses above this upper bound (LongP) were excluded from computation. These occurred when the tape to be analyzed was stopped and speech ended, yet the computer was not simultaneously shut down. Verifying this are the oscillogram records which visually display no speech pause of this length.

In all recording sessions, an artificial non-linguistic pause was introduced whenever E presented a new picture to S. This took an average of 2.5 seconds for each individual subject. This is compensated for in the program by the equation

$$\text{Ave} = \frac{(\text{Sum} - 95)}{(\text{Num} - 38)}$$

This methodology outlined here succinctly deals with the many problems encountered in the measurements of silent intervals in continuous speech. It also avoids the tedious and impressionistic approaches which have very often plagued researchers in this area.

Maclay and Osgood (1959) had basically no criterion at all for an unfilled pause. Levin and Silverman (1965) point out the difficulties involved:

> The first review of the tapes was for the express purpose of timing the pauses. This was done by a stop watch at least twice for each pause. Pauses less than a second in duration were simply noted since the accuracy of using a stop watch did not permit greater precision than one second. Pauses longer than one second were timed to the closest second. (p. 72)

Goldman-Eisler (1958b) employed a pen-recorder which traced the sound-impulses on a magnetic tape into a visual record. This allowed her to mark pauses down to 100 msec. Accurate though this record is, only a small body of speech data can economically be analyzed.

Another mechanical method was proposed by Boomer (1965). While speech was being tape recorded, a simultaneous oscillogram was made in order to find silent pauses. Every 30 seconds an automatic timer marked signals on both the oscillogram and on the tape. This aided in matching these records with the typescripts. The threshold for an unfilled pause was any duration above 200 msec and was marked on the transcript from the visual record.

Although the computer programs very effectively measured pauses and performed other analyses of the data, thus allowing LARGE corpora to be handled, there still would remain the very laborious task of locating and marking UPs in written transcripts. It would be necessary, therefore, to employ the use of a stop watch in order to manually locate the silences. Once a criterion for what constitutes an unfilled pause would be established, each tape would be played back at the original recording speed and when a pause would occur a slanted line (/) would be inserted on the typescript.

III

TWO HESITATION VARIABLES: FILLED AND UNFILLED PAUSE

The problem of what constitutes an Unfilled Pause is obvious, *i.e.*, we have to ask what criterion has to be satisfied in order that a silent hesitation can be classified as an Unfilled Pause. Maclay and Osgood (1959) were quite casual in this regard when they stated that:

> UP has two major forms: silence of unusual length and non-phonemic lengthening of phonemes. This is necessarily a matter of judgment on the part of listeners (here, the authors) familiar with the pace and style of a particular speaker. What may be clearly noted as an instance of Unfilled Pause for one speaker would not be so judged for another speaker, say, with a slower rate of delivery. (p. 24)

This definition undoubtedly lacks objectivity and is outright useless because 'the pace and style of a particular speaker' appeals to the previous history of an organism; and for present purposes this type of information—how an aphasic patient used language premorbidly—is not available to the experimenter.

The second computer program outlined above proved to be of more objective usefulness because it provides median scores of pause lengths. Table 1 lists the median pause lengths for Task 1.

In checking the print-outs of the pause-length analyses of the aphasic population, the high values obtained are immediately apparent. Thus mean scores would turn out to be quite misleading (although average scores were part of the body of statistical information computed by the frequency distribution program). In this study averaged data might conceal pause length discrepancies because it is highly skewed as a result of the occurrence of very long pause durations. In addition, taking the mean over a group of subjects may obscure final results. Median values, on the other hand, provide here subtler insights and are of greater sensitivity to the data.

TABLE 1

Median Pause Durations of Aphasics and Normals
(N = 16)

Subjects	Medians (sec.)	Subjects	Medians (sec.)
A1	1.38	N1	1.20
A2	1.04	N2	1.04
A3	.88	N3	.84
A4	1.76	N4	.70
A5	1.16	N5	.88
A6	.84	N6	1.02
A7	1.24	N7	.58
A8	1.82	N8	.72

As can be seen from Table 1, the median range of pause duration for the aphasics went from .84 seconds to 1.82 seconds and for the normals from .58 seconds to 1.20 seconds. Taken together, the medians of the aphasics cluster around 1.26 seconds and those of the normals around .87 seconds. That amounts to an almost 40 % difference between the two populations and therefore is highly significant. This motivated our decision to establish one second as the threshold for UP. This choice of a baseline value is satisfactory in that it was arrived at empirically and not postulated in any preconceived way. It is also in keeping with a result of a study published by Hargreaves and Starkweather (1959). Their duration tabulator agreed with human judges for silent hesitations of one second and up. Therefore, they marked one second as the lower bound for this type of pause.

In addition to the measurements of the lengths of the non-speech intervals, an analysis of the locations of both pausal types was performed. Maclay and Osgood worked with the Fries (1952) set of major form-classes. This classification system comprises four part-of-speech classes, roughly relating to nouns, verbs, adjectives and adverbs (in that order) of traditional grammar and fifteen function word groups. This frame of reference seemed also sufficiently acceptable for this investigation in order to determine the environment of the two types of hesitation.[1] These two changes in nomenclature were incorporated: the four structural word classes are called LEXICAL and all function word groups are referred to as NON-LEXICAL.

However, during the analysis, the Fries framework turned out to be inadequate at times. He did not deal with proper nouns or with *to* as infinitive marker of a verb. Consequently they were not included in this study. Also two-morpheme adverbs like *of course* and *at least* were not treated in his book. On the other hand, for certain items it was difficult or impossible to establish membership in any of the given classes because of neologisms occurring in aphasic speech, except by projection or arbitrarily:

A2 "... they're /[2] [ə] / *sweelin'* down".
A4: "I like music and [ə] / they [ə] / *cupka.*"
A6: "They are got [ə] / *stattered.*"

[1] Since Fries' data consisted of recorded telephone conversations, it shared with the data of the present paper the characteristics of spontaneous speech. Fries did not analyse rehearsed test sentences and therefore omitted any kind of punctuation in his transcripts and in doing so side-stepped problems of suprasegmentals. Furthermore, the classes are defined strictly on syntactic grounds and not semantically.

As regards the essential distinction between *utterances* and *sentences*, Lehrer (1968) follows Chomsky's (*e.g.*, 1965) original observations when she comments: "An utterance is a linguistic event, something actually uttered by a speaker in some situation. Utterances are for physiological and psychological reasons limited in length and complexity. By contrast, sentences are theoretical elements in a theory of language and are not so limited. Many utterances contain various 'mistakes,' i.e., repetitions, hesitations, noises, uncompleted items, etc." (p. 85)

[2] Slanted line indicates UP.

Again, any occurrence of a pause preceding such an item was not counted. If two or more FPs occurred in a row, they were counted as one occurrence. If both a FP and an UP preceded an item, they were both scored as one event of each pause type but if the sequence was / [ə] then the UP was not considered in connection with an item following [ə]. If the UP happened to be located between the two components of a compound noun, it was marked as a pause before a Class 1 word (*e.g.*, bow / tie).

The analysis of the transcripts concerned the positions of both pause types in regard to linguistic form classes. Task 1 and Task 2 of each subject were analysed four times, namely FP preceding lexical items, FP before non-lexical items, UP preceding lexical items, and UP before non-lexical items. This yielded numerical results for the four lexical classes and fifteen non-lexical groups shown in the Tables 2 and 3.

According to the Maclay/Osgood hypothesis, the figures obtained for UP in the lexical categories should be greater than those in the non-lexical categories. Table 4 displays the ratios between the two types of pauses.

The ratios obtained for A2, A6, A8, and A9, as shown in Table 4, give evidence that the above mentioned premise can hardly be upheld since actually only 60 % of the aphasics bear it out. Among the normals, much of the same is obvious: N3, N5, N6, N7, N8 either display near-equal values (close similarity between UP and FP) or refute the hypothesis outright.

The other corollary of this hypothesis states that the occurrences of FP preceding non-lexical items are more frequent than those preceding lexical items. Table 5 presents the relevant ratios that hold between the two pause types.

Except for one case, N7, both populations' figures point to the exact opposite of the presumed tenet.

The data in Table 6 tabulate ratios of both hesitation types for Task 2.

The findings clearly indicate further that the behavior of filled and unfilled pauses in regard to syntactic environment is different from the Maclay and Osgood predictions. Among the aphasics only A1, A3, A7, and A10 and among the normals only N2 and N4 support the asserted distribution.

Table 7 presents comparable ratios to Table 5 for the two variables as obtained in Task 2.

TABLE 2

Distribution of Filled and Unfilled Pause by the Form Classes Following Pause (Task 1)

Subject	Environment	FP	UP	Subject	Environment	FP	UP
A1	Lexical	1	147	N1	Lexical	7	120
	Non-Lexical	1	136		Non-Lexical	5	200
A2	Lexical	168	163	N2	Lexical	8	34
	Non-Lexical	113	133		Non-Lexical	0	40
A3	Lexical	122	228	N3	Lexical	35	38
	Non-Lexical	72	201		Non-Lexical	20	36
A4	Lexical	57	150	N4	Lexical	6	33
	Non-Lexical	49	172		Non-Lexical	6	42
A5	Lexical	114	135	N5	Lexical	52	53
	Non-Lexical	70	157		Non-Lexical	50	60
A6	Lexical	82	54	N6	Lexical	75	53
	Non-Lexical	61	60		Non-Lexical	58	122
A7	Lexical	16	124	N7	Lexical	47	18
	Non-Lexical	11	102		Non-Lexical	13	8
A8	Lexical	89	77	N8	Lexical	38	34
	Non-Lexical	54	172		Non-Lexical	16	39
A9	Lexical	180	162	N9	Lexical	34	117
	Non-Lexical	176	245		Non-Lexical	22	164
A10	Lexical	30	78	N10	Lexical	24	60
	Non-Lexical	8	113		Non-Lexical	7	48

TABLE 3

Distribution of Filled and Unfilled Pause by the Form Classes Following Pause (Task 2)

Subject	Environment	FP	UP	Subject	Environment	FP	UP
A1	Lexical	7	54	N1	Lexical	28	25
	Non-Lexical	8	32		Non-Lexical	26	42
A2	Lexical	89	52	N2	Lexical	2	17
	Non-Lexical	45	61		Non-Lexical	2	23
A3	Lexical	16	52	N3	Lexical	34	26
	Non-Lexical	15	37		Non-Lexical	15	27
A4	Lexical	78	55	N4	Lexical	4	18
	Non-Lexical	43	84		Non-Lexical	4	35
A5	Lexical	74	29	N5	Lexical	37	16
	Non-Lexical	67	46		Non-Lexical	38	16
A6	Lexical	71	14	N6	Lexical	71	21
	Non-Lexical	22	7		Non-Lexical	41	38
A7	Lexical	37	94	N7	Lexical	15	9
	Non-Lexical	18	81		Non-Lexical	8	5
A8	Lexical	52	49	N8	Lexical	45	18
	Non-Lexical	43	49		Non-Lexical	20	27
A9	Lexical	59	59	N9	Lexical	51	25
	Non-Lexical	70	113		Non-Lexical	23	17
A10	Lexical	30	37	N10	Lexical	32	11
	Non-Lexical	23	58		Non-Lexical	11	18

The total amount of pausal occurrences (both UP and FP) was less in Task 2 than in Task 1. This can be attributed to the fact that the speaker took less time to answer E's questions, *i.e.*, the speech output was decreased from the picture describing task. The number of pauses is a function of verbal output.

TABLE 4

Ratios of UP to FP (Lexical) Task 1

Subjects	R=UP(L):FP(L)	Subjects	R=UP(L):FP(L)
A1	147.00:1	N1	17.14:1
A2	.97:1	N2	4.25:1
A3	1.87:1	N3	1.08:1
A4	2.63:1	N4	5.50:1
A5	1.18:1	N5	1.01:1
A6	.66:1	N6	.71:1
A7	7.75:1	N7	.38:1
A8	.87:1	N8	.89:1
A9	.90:1	N9	3.44:1
A10	2.60:1	N10	2.50:1

TABLE 5

Ratios of FP to UP (Non-Lexical) Task 1

Subjects	R=FP(NL):UP(NL)	Subjects	R=FP(NL):UP(NL)
A1	.01:1	N1	.03:1
A2	.85:1	N2	0:1
A3	.36:1	N3	.56:1
A4	.28:1	N4	.14:1
A5	.44:1	N5	.83:1
A6	1.02:1	N6	.48:1
A7	.11:1	N7	1.63:1
A8	.31:1	N8	.41:1
A9	.72:1	N9	.13:1
A10	.07:1	N10	.15:1

But also in the free speech sample, as can be seen from Table 7, only A5 and A6, and N5, N7, and N9 are in support of the Maclay-Osgood observation whereas all other subjects differ significantly

TABLE 6

Ratios of UP to FP (Lexical) Task 2

Subjects	R=UP(L):FP(L)	Subjects	R=UP(L):FP(L)
A1	7.71:1	N1	.89:1
A2	.58:1	N2	8.50:1
A3	3.25:1	N3	.76:1
A4	.71:1	N4	4.50:1
A5	.39:1	N5	.43:1
A6	.20:1	N6	.30:1
A7	2.54:1	N7	.60:1
A8	.94:1	N8	.40:1
A9	1.00:1	N9	.49:1
A10	1.23:1	N10	.34:1

TABLE 7

Ratios of FP to UP (Non-Lexical) Task 2

Subjects	R=FP(NL):UP(NL)	Subjects	R=FP(NL):UP(NL)
A1	.25:1	N1	.62:1
A2	.74:1	N2	.09:1
A3	.41:1	N3	.56:1
A4	.51:1	N4	.11:1
A5	1.46:1	N5	2.38:1
A6	3.14:1	N6	1.08:1
A7	.22:1	N7	1.60:1
A8	.88:1	N8	.74:1
A9	.62:1	N9	1.35:1
A10	.40:1	N10	.61:1

from it. As a matter of fact, the data indicate (Table 5 and Table 7) that filled pauses occupy considerably less the position before non-lexical items than unfilled pauses do.

TABLE 8

Ratios of FP to Lexical vs. Non-Lexical Items (Task 1)

Subjects	R=FP(NL):FP(L)	Subjects	R=FP(NL):FP(L)
A1	1.00:1	N1	.71:1
A2	.67:1	N2	0:1
A3	.59:1	N3	.57:1
A4	.86:1	N4	1.00:1
A5	.61:1	N5	.96:1
A6	.74:1	N6	.77:1
A7	.69:1	N7	.28:1
A8	.61:1	N8	.42:1
A9	.98:1	N9	.65:1
A10	.27:1	N10	.29:1

TABLE 9

Ratios of UP to Lexical vs. Non-Lexical Items (Task 1)

Subjects	R=UP(L):UP(NL)	Subjects	R=UP(L):UP(NL)
A1	1.08:1	N1	.60:1
A2	1.23:1	N2	.85:1
A3	1.13:1	N3	1.06:1
A4	.87:1	N4	.79:1
A5	.86:1	N5	.88:1
A6	.90:1	N6	.43:1
A7	1.19:1	N7	2.25:1
A8	.45:1	N8	.87:1
A9	.66:1	N9	.71:1
A10	.69:1	N10	1.25:1

The distributions of filled and unfilled pauses were checked further in regard to lexical vs. non-lexical items for both Tasks based on the data of Tables 2 and 3. The next four tables contain the ratios of FP and UP to lexical vs. non-lexical items (Tables 8-11).

TABLE 10

Ratios of FP to Lexical vs. Non-Lexical Items (Task 2)

Subjects	R=FP(NL):FP(L)	Subjects	R=FP(NL):FP(L)
A1	1.14:1	N1	.93:1
A2	.51:1	N2	1.00:1
A3	.94:1	N3	.44:1
A4	.55:1	N4	1.00:1
A5	.91:1	N5	1.03:1
A6	.31:1	N6	.58:1
A7	.49:1	N7	.53:1
A8	.83:1	N8	.44:1
A9	1.19:1	N9	.45:1
A10	.77:1	N10	.34:1

TABLE 11

Ratios of UP to Lexical vs. Non-Lexical Items (Task 2)

Subjects	R=UP(L):UP(NL)	Subjects	R=UP(L):UP(NL)
A1	1.69:1	N1	.60:1
A2	.85:1	N2	.74:1
A3	1.41:1	N3	.96:1
A4	.65:1	N4	.51:1
A5	.63:1	N5	1.00:1
A6	2.00:1	N6	.55:1
A7	1.16:1	N7	1.80:1
A8	1.00:1	N8	.67:1
A9	.52:1	N9	1.47:1
A10	.64:1	N10	.61:1

Our results clearly suggest that the premise establishing a non-random distribution of these two hesitation phenomena in respect to form classes can by no means be justified. Especially the variable filled pause refutes the claim stating that it occurs more frequently before non-lexical than before lexical items since 38 ratios out of a total of 40 negate this position (Tables 8 and 10). As for the unfilled pauses, the magnitude of deviance is less: 29 ratios out of 40 contradict the Maclay/Osgood conclusions. However, the 11 ratios bearing it out are too weak a basis for generalization of this kind.

The preceding four tables also illustrate that there was no difference either in the ratios of the two hesitation types or in the ratios in regard to lexical vs. non-lexical items when the two tasks were compared. This holds for both experimental populations.

In the same paper (1959), the authors write:

> Since, as Fries notes, there are many more members (alternatives) in his lexical classes than in his function word classes, we should expect pauses of both types to occur more frequently before lexical words than before function words. Table 5 provides a test of this hypothesis. According to chance, it is assumed, pauses would occur equally in each possible position; actually, both Filled Pauses and Unfilled Pauses are found to occur significantly more frequently before lexical words than before function words. (p. 32)

An inspection of Tables 2 and 3 shows this to be the case for filled pauses (with minor exceptions) but the data is not in agreement for unfilled pauses. In the few cases of silent hesitations that confirm the above hypothesis, they are found, of all places, among the aphasics. Although the lexical class as the open form class definitely is greater in size than the closed non-lexical form class, it does not follow that unfilled pauses precede the former more frequently.

On the basis of the scoring sheets that list the numerical results of the Friesian classes, an analysis was performed as to what classes had the most entries. This covers both populations and both Tasks. There were 77 incidents of Class 1 ("nouns") and only 3 exceptions. Those were all Class 2 ("verbs"), all found in normals, all in Task 1, and 2 in the UP variable, 1 in the FP variable.

Group A (the class of all determiners) occurred 41 times, with 10 inconclusive scores and 29 exceptions to Group A, of which

TABLE 12

Form Classes with Highest Frequencies Following both Pausal Types

		A1		
TASK 1	FP/lexical	class 1	UP/lexical	class 1
	FP/non-lexical	Group E	UP/non-lexical	Group A
TASK 2	FP/lexical	class 1	UP/lexical	class 1
	FP/non-lexical	Group A	UP/non-lexical	Group A
		N1		
TASK 1	FP/lexical	class 1	UP/lexical	class 1
	FP/non-lexical	%[1]	UP/non-lexical	Group F
TASK 2	FP/lexical	class 1	UP/lexical	class 1
	FP/non-lexical	Group A	UP/non-lexical	Group J

		A2		
TASK 1	FP/lexical	class 1	UP/lexical	class 1
	FP/non-lexical	Group A	UP/non-lexical	Group A
TASK 2	FP/lexical	class 1	UP/lexical	class 1
	FP/non-lexical	Group A	UP/non-lexical	Group A
		N2		
TASK 1	FP/lexical	class 1	UP/lexical	class 1
	FP/non-lexical	none	UP/non-lexical	Group E
TASK 2	FP/lexical	class 1	UP/lexical	class 1
	FP/non-lexical	%	UP/non-lexical	Group J

		A3		
TASK 1	FP/lexical	class 1	UP/lexical	class 1
	FP/non-lexical	Group A	UP/non-lexical	Group J
TASK 2	FP/lexical	class 1	UP/lexical	class 1
	FP/non-lexical	%	UP/non-lexical	Group J
		N3		
TASK 1	FP/lexical	class 2	UP/lexical	class 1
	FP/non-lexical	Group A	UP/non-lexical	Group A
TASK 2	FP/lexical	class 1	UP/lexical	class 1
	FP/non-lexical	Group A	UP/non-lexical	Group A

[1] % indicates a tie between two or several classes.

A4

TASK 1	FP/lexical	class 1	UP/lexical	class 1
	FP/non-lexical	Group A	UP/non-lexical	Group A
TASK 2	FP/lexical	class 1	UP/lexical	class 1
	FP/non-lexical	Group A	UP/non-lexical	Group E

N4

TASK 1	FP/lexical	class 1	UP/lexical	class 1
	FP/non-lexical	%	UP/non-lexical	Group E
TASK 2	FP/lexical	class 1	UP/lexical	class 1
	FP/non-lexical	%	UP/non-lexical	Group J

A5

TASK 1	FP/lexical	class 1	UP/lexical	class 1
	FP/non-lexical	Group A	UP/non-lexical	Group J
TASK 2	FP/lexical	class 1	UP/lexical	class 1
	FP/non-lexical	Group A	UP/non-lexical	Group J

N5

TASK 1	FP/lexical	class 1	UP/lexical	class 1
	FP/non-lexical	Group A	UP/non-lexical	Group A
TASK 2	FP/lexical	class 1	UP/lexical	class 1
	FP/non-lexical	Group A	UP/non-lexical	Group J

A6

TASK 1	FP/lexical	class 1	UP/lexical	class 1
	FP/non-lexical	Group A	UP/non-lexical	Group A
TASK 2	FP/lexical	class 1	UP/lexical	class 1
	FP/non-lexical	Group A	UP/non-lexical	Group A

N6

TASK 1	FP/lexical	class 1	UP/lexical	class 2
	FP/non-lexical	Group A	UP/non-lexical	Group J
TASK 2	FP/lexical	class 1	UP/lexical	class 1
	FP/non-lexical	Group A	UP/non-lexical	Group E

A7

TASK 1	FP/lexical	class 1	UP/lexical	class 1
	FP/non-lexical	Group A	UP/non-lexical	Group J
TASK 2	FP/lexical	class 1	UP/lexical	class 1
	FP/non-lexical	Group J	UP/non-lexical	Group J

N7

TASK 1	FP/lexical	class 1	UP/lexical	class 2
	FP/non-lexical	Group A	UP/non-lexical	Group A
TASK 2	FP/lexical	class 1	UP/lexical	class 1
	FP/non-lexical	Group A	UP/non-lexical	Group J

A8

TASK 1	FP/lexical	class 1	UP/lexical	class 1
	FP/non-lexical	Group K	UP/non-lexical	Group K
TASK 2	FP/lexical	class 1	UP/lexical	class 1
	FP/non-lexical	Group K	UP/non-lexical	Group K

N8

TASK 1	FP/lexical	class 1	UP/lexical	class 1
	FP/non-lexical	Group A	UP/non-lexical	%
TASK 2	FP/lexical	class 1	UP/lexical	class 1
	FP/non-lexical	Group A	UP/non-lexical	Group J

A9

TASK 1	FP/lexical	class 1	UP/lexical	class 1
	FP/non-lexical	Group A	UP/non-lexical	Group A
TASK 2	FP/lexical	class 1	UP/lexical	class 1
	FP/non-lexical	Group K	UP/non-lexical	%

N9

TASK 1	FP/lexical	class 1	UP/lexical	class 1
	FP/non-lexical	Group A	UP/non-lexical	Group A
TASK 2	FP/lexical	class 1	UP/lexical	class 1
	FP/non-lexical	%	UP/non-lexical	Group J

A10

TASK 1	FP/lexical FP/non-lexical	class 1 Group A	UP/lexical UP/non-lexical	class 1 Group A
TASK 2	FP/lexical FP/non-lexical	class 1 Group A	UP/lexical UP/non-lexical	class 1 %

N10

TASK 1	FP/lexical FP/non-lexical	class 1 Group F	UP/lexical UP/non-lexical	class 1 Group K
TASK 2	FP/lexical FP/non-lexical	class 1 Group A	UP/lexical UP/non-lexical	class 1 Group J

14 were found in the aphasics and 15 in normals. The exceptions divide themselves in the following way:

16: Group J
6: Group K
5: Group E
2: Group F

Twenty-three of them (9 in Task 1, 14 in Task 2) were in UP; 6 in FP (3 in Task 1, 3 in Task 2).

The pause type filled pause contained 27 instances of Group A plus 6 exceptions, whereas the pause type unfilled pause contained 14 instances of Group A plus 23 exceptions. Thus the latter variable is more often associated with non-lexical items. This conclusion is further proof that it cannot be maintained that UP precedes more often lexical items than non-lexical ones.

In dealing with hesitancy in Task 1, two quantities have to be taken into consideration: total pause time ($T_{(P)}$) and total speaking time. The former was one of the parameters provided by the computer frequency distribution program. Goldman-Eisler (1961b) expressed the reverse of fluency, hesitancy, as follows:

There are various ways of expressing the degree of hesitation in speech. If duration of pauses is the basic quantity it must be related to the length of the utterance whose degree of hesitation (or hesitancy) is to be measured. In any speech sequence pause and speech periods usually alternate in an irregular and seemingly unsystematic fashion. Naturally, pauses accumulate and with increasing length of utterance the total pause time also increases. Hesitancy is therefore a ratio of pause time to speech time, if by speech we refer to vocal action only. (p. 167)

The basic problem here is what measure should be used to account for TOTAL SPEAKING TIME. Of course, all kinds of criteria could be advanced, taken from several linguistic frameworks, in order to determine how and what to count in written transcripts of recorded vocal productions. For example, the corpus of each subject could be analyzed in terms of ICs or on the basis of derivations within the transformational-generative grammar model or simply statistically with the type/token ratio.

If, however, total speaking time is considered to be the total number of words in the corpus, then we are immediately faced with the question of finding a consistent criterion of that elusive linguistic unit, the word. Incidentally, we are focusing on the total number of words in the ENTIRE corpus, not on the number of words per utterance since the latter's boundaries have been assigned subjectively on the typescripts, dealing with SPOKEN data.

There has been a prolonged linguistic dispute, often bordering on polemic, about this unit of speech. Quite often a word is defined as that unit which ends when the space bar is depressed while typing, *i.e.*, the basis for decision is taken from written or printed materials. This blank space rule is of course erroneous since nobody speaks in printed words. Furthermore, words in speech do not occur in isolation but rather as a continuum. That is why no linguist would propose a definition of a word in purely phonetic terms. Thus far criteria have included lexical-statistic, morphological, syntactic or semantic considerations. And yet linguists have not been reluctant to establish such notions as word-initial, word-medial and word-final in descriptive analysis. There is no doubt about a word-initial position as being a valid discrimination, just in case it is also UTTERANCE-initial. But the other two are a matter of juncture, stress and similar suprasegmental features and are difficult to isolate in a running speech sample.

Greenberg (1965) points out the arbitrary nature of this utterance segment:

The word as a unit occupies a paradoxical situation in present-day linguistic science. Such a unit, roughly coinciding with the usage of the term in every day language and in the discourse of sciences other than linguistics, is actually employed as a fundamental dividing line between the two levels of morphological (infra-word) constructions and syntactic (supra-word) constructions. Yet no generally accepted and satisfactory definition exists, and some linguists deny validity of the word altogether, relegating it to folk-linguistics. Others believe that the word must be defined separately for each language and that there are probably languages to which the concept is inapplicable. Some define the word in phonological terms, as when a word in Czech is defined as a sequence with stress on its initial syllable. Other definitions depend on the distribution of meaningful units and may be qualified as morphological or grammatical. (p. 66)

In their discussion of juncture phenomena Trager and Smith (1957) propose the term PHONEMIC WORD by stating:

A phonemic phrase having no plus juncture (and consequently no secondary stresses) will be called a Phonemic Word; it is the limiting case. These terms have, it must be noted, no connotation whatsoever of morphology; they are purely phonological. (p. 50)

This unit was adopted here as the basis for counting the number of words in each subject's corpus. It is intuitively satisfactory inasmuch as only phonological considerations are decisive in this type of analysis. Thus it is very much in keeping with the scope of this study and most appropriate to the type of data being analyzed.

Most recent work in transformational phonology again raises the question about the formal properties of the unit, WORD. In dealing with formative boundaries Chomsky and Halle (1968) seem to support the notion "phonemic word" when they observe:

Expressions such as *differing*, *ringing*, *metalanguage*, *establishment* are single words from the point of view of the phonological rules, and the definition "word" must certainly be designed so as to express this fact. But convention (115) will assign an interval # boundary in these expressions because they contain the elements *differ*, *ring*, *language*, *establish*, each of which belongs to a lexical category. Thus convention (115) gives the forms:

(116) (a) [V # [V # differ #] V ing #] V
(b) [V # [V # ring #] V ing #] V

(c) [N# meta [N# language #] N#] N
(d) [N# [V# establish #] V ment #] N

... Nevertheless, we want to regard the full forms of (116) as single words. (p. 367)

The dropping of internal occurrence of # in certain positions corresponds to the definition of phonemic word, a phonemic phrase without plus junctures.

The following procedure for the phonemic word count was undertaken. In addition to the written transcript, the respective tape of each S was also played back in order to ensure that the scoring was not solely based on the typed text, which is based on the alphabet and therefore biased. Working with both these records, the visual and the auditory, turned out to be successful. Inflectional verb endings like the *-n't* of *don't* and *aren't* were scored as one unit. So were noun-verb contractions like *I'm*, *I'd* or instances of *that's*. Furthermore, some subjects pronounce the pronouns *them* ~ *'em*, *her* ~ *'er* with weak stress in utterances such as "I like 'em". This manifestation ['laykəm] was also counted as one unit. Included also were word repetitions. Word fragments and all other kinds of non-linguistic noise were ignored. Table 13 gives the relevant statistical data on hesitancy.

Comparing the entries of this table, three dimensions of difference are noticeable that sharply distinguish the aphasic patients from the normal subjects, *viz.*, the former have silent hesitations of longer durations, pause more often and display reduced verbal productivity when compared to both total pause and total speaking times. The aphasics' silence intervals are often triple in length in comparison to the total speaking time of a recording session. Further evidence for these temporal increments from the normals is apparent from Table 14, tabulating the mean pause lengths of both populations.

Our findings are hard to dismiss because of the fairly objective nature in which the data was analysed. They are inconsistent with the results of earlier investigations and thus supersede them. In general, it can be said that both hesitation variables are not patterned in speech as previously interpreted. They do occur in a non-random systematic fashion but the distributions cannot be said to exist so definitively or in such absolute terms.

The analysis fails to show a difference in distribution of filled and unfilled pauses in regard to lexical and non-lexical items. It also could not be verified that BOTH FP and UP precede lexical items more frequently; only for the variable FP was the data in agreement.

TABLE 13

Relative Hesitancy = Pause/Speech Ratio (N=16)

Sub-jects	SUM sec.	Phonemic word count	Sub-jects	SUM sec.	Phonemic word count
A1	SUM[a] 1839.56 NUM[b] 721	787	N1	SUM 1324.16 NUM 742	2596
A2	SUM 2433.68 NUM 1343	2169	N2	SUM 438.42 NUM 237	1937
A3	SUM 1942.32 NUM 1857	3614	N3	SUM 424.50 NUM 333	1095
A4	SUM 2006.38 NUM 646	1333	N4	SUM 506.30 NUM 429	2559
A5	SUM 1798.34 NUM 837	2240	N5	SUM 579.16 NUM 535	2654
A6	SUM 1203.66 NUM 949	1661	N6	SUM 620.24 NUM 442	1645
A7	SUM 1476.32 NUM 603	1983	N7	SUM 408.52 NUM 437	2156
A8	SUM 2531.28 NUM 718	1572	N8	SUM 693.06 NUM 608	2549

[a] SUM: total length of pause periods in seconds
[b] NUM: total number of pauses exceeding threshold value

TABLE 14

Mean Pause Durations of Aphasics and Normals (N=16)

Subjects	Means sec.	Subjects	Means sec.
A1	2.55	N1	1.75
A2	1.79	N2	1.72
A3	1.02	N3	1.12
A4	3.14	N4	1.05
A5	2.13	N5	.97
A6	1.22	N6	1.30
A7	2.44	N7	.79
A8	3.58	N8	1.05

On the other hand, both the aphasics and the normals in this study were externally consistent with one another in regard to the occurrences of the hesitation types in relation to form classes. That is to say, the aphasics both as a group and as individuals displayed about the same patterning in their pausing behavior as the matched subjects. No aphasia-specific deficit was observed, although this at first had been anticipated. It therefore has to be concluded that they do not differ qualitatively from the normals.

The type of distributions obtained in Task 1 were the same as those of Task 2, although the eliciting stimulus of the former was visual, the one in the latter auditory.

However, the degree of deviance in the patients clearly showed itself in three fundamental parameters of this study: median scores, total lengths of pauses in relation to the amount of verbal output, and number of pauses. Therefore one could say that the speech pathology is directly reflected in the frequency and durational aspects of unfilled pauses. And this makes for a quantitative difference. Thus we regard length-of-pause as a definite dimension of deviance in aphasic speech.

IV

CONCLUDING REMARKS

The general conclusions drawn from this study are of two kinds.

First of all, considering the wide variety of causes of the cortical insults among the aphasics, they all shared in the language deficit known as ANOMIA or 'word-finding' difficulty (inability to name objects or events); some evidenced this to a lesser or greater degree than others. Word-finding problems also occur in the speech of normals, though only sporadically and not as consistently as in the verbal repertoire of an aphasic. This impairment alone, which is still a residual problem long after the state of spontaneous recovery has passed and even after speech therapy has started, would make one assume that it would probably have an effect on the overall physical structure of utterances although anomia is particularly related to the noun class. Moreover, the impediment in aphasic verbal behavior was apparent in some patients' elliptical syntax, particularly the omission of certain classes of non-lexical items. This too was considered a factor in the breakdown of the normal speech process, resulting in fragmented utterances, and would with all likelihood have consequences for pausal distributions. That is to say, deviant distributions of both the spoken hesitations and the silent gaps in the flow of spontaneous speech, which all control an utterance, were anticipated. However, the foregoing analysis demonstrates no qualitative differences from normal controls of this very elementary feature of speech, pausing. This observation, in its way, supports the conclusions of a study by Carson, Carson and Tikofsky (1968) of a different area of the aphasic syndrome. These authors conducted four different kinds of experiments on nonverbal performance tasks in order to test the effect of learning on subsequent performance trials. They provide this summary:

> Aphasics showed significant regularities in their ability to learn new tasks, to retain their skill over time, and to handle a wide range of complexity in stimulus material. Characteristics which distinguished them from normals were their slower speed and frequently their lower level of attainment. They did not distinguish themselves as a group from normals by inability to perform on any of the difficult experimental tasks. (p. 110)

Secondly, the statistical analysis of the spontaneous speech data by electronic pause detection and measuring techniques yielded marked quantitative differences in the aphasic population. The quantity of time that elapsed when the speech stream was interrupted increased significantly. This finding was expected to begin with, and came as no surprise as an aphasic may punctuate the flow of speech by prolonged intervals for all or some of the following reasons in spontaneous speech:

(1) He may be anomic, *i.e.*, it takes a concentrated effort in the production of the appropriate item on the part of the speaker.
(2) He may process a pictorial stimulus more slowly resulting in increased latencies. Each picture constitutes a behavioral episode and after each one has been described there will necessarily occur initial delays before the next one.
(3) He may encode a phrase of an utterance more slowly because of reduced availability of syntactic sequencing of individual elements in the speech process but also because of the condition stated in (1). These factors handicap the facility of initiating speech.

In addition to these conclusions that account for the non-fluency of aphasic speech, it can also be said that there is no distinctive functional difference between a vocalized hesitation and a silent pause. Both filled and unfilled pauses exhibit close distributions in their occurrence preceding Class 1 words and Group A words. A further conclusion is apparent: The great number of unfilled pauses before non-lexical items appears to suggest that subjects, both aphasics and normals, self-interrupt the vocal/verbal stream considerably to select these items, as well as before lexical items. This fact differs from the proposal (*e.g.*, Goodglass, 1962) made in connection with the agrammatic syndrome in aphasia that considers only lexical items as the key selections to be made by the speaker and therefore assumes that at those locations points of hesitation are to be found. Thus both types of hesitations tended to occur in places of lexical (anomia) and structural (cf. above) points of non-fluency concerning the following word.

The most striking question raised by this study about the Maclay-Osgood findings is this: what factors account for the dissimilar distributions of hesitation phenomena between their NORMAL subjects and our NORMAL subjects? That even the normals in this study did not support these authors' findings was unexpected here. One could hardly attribute the difference to idiosyncratic features in a speaker's verbal behavior although pausal patterns are sometimes a conditioned personality characteristic. However, the overall magnitude of disagreement rules this out. Rather, clues to the non-confirming results are provided by the conditions of their experiment. The experimental population was biased inasmuch as it consisted solely of male professionals who served as informants. The subjects of this study, on the other hand, were more representative as they were selected from many social and educational backgrounds. Secondly, their experimental setting for data acquisition was confined to a conference-type discussion on highly specialized topics whereas eight out of ten of the normal control subject sessions for this work were conducted in the subjects' homes. This environment plus the stimulus material could be considered more conducive to the elicitation of a sample of spontaneous speech.

It also seems that the sample chosen for the analysis of filled and unfilled pauses relative to lexical vs. non-lexical items was too limited. The investigators took "a sample of sixteen word sequences or frames that occurred relatively frequently in the data ... for detailed analysis." (p. 31) No further defining criteria for this choice are given. However, this analysis covered very large linguistic corpora in their entirety without isolating particular phrases. Goldman-Eisler's (1958b) results were in keeping with those of Maclay and Osgood with regard to the observation that unfilled pauses were immediately followed by lexical items. But the samples of her analysis were linguistically quite artificial and unrealistic since she selected for the experiment only the rarer sentences that do not contain any deviations from well-formedness.

Finally, when Maclay and Osgood comment "that Filled Pause is RELATIVELY more likely to appear before function words, while Unfilled Pause is RELATIVELY more likely to appear before lexical words ..." (p. 33, emphasis mine.), they were wise in their choice of the term RELATIVE inasmuch as it is not feasible, judging from our findings, to make an absolute claim regarding the above distributions. In fact, upon analyzing our data it can be stated that the distributions are even more varied and relative than their Table 5 (which only lists two examples) indicates. Rather their later position verifying that "these two types of pauses are not in complementary distribution linguistically, since either type CAN occur in any position where the other occurs and does so frequently" (p. 39) seemingly refutes their basic leanings toward a 'relative' PATTERN of hesitations which they call statistically significant.

There is one more clue to be mentioned in this discussion. In checking the speech sample (p. 25) in regard to location of FP and UP it was found that indeed there were five cases of FP preceding non-lexical items. However, there were also six cases where FP was in positions before lexical items. If this can occur in even such a short sample, one wonders how valid the position later taken can be justified.

Turning now to some of the theoretical implications contained in the results, there are some interesting insights to note when focusing on the data of Table 12. It showed that both hesitation pauses had occurrences of highest frequencies either before Class 1 members or Group A members, *i.e.*, their position is either pre-Noun or pre-Noun Phrase. In our body of data 50% of the nouns, conservatively estimated, were subject personal pronouns, which according to Fries were grouped with the lexical Form Class 1.

Nouns were distributed throughout the utterances and occurred in subject, object, and predicate nominative positions. Utterances with single nouns following a non-speech interval were more frequent than those with an extended noun phrase. When a pause was located in pre-NP position, the NP, made up of D + N, was manifested as one unit. Only very infrequently were there cases like Group A — pause — Class 1 (/ the / patio). The majority of all noun phrases consisted of two elements, D and N, and there were hardly any with the shape Group A — Class 3 — Class 1.

At times there was evidence of fragmented utterance partials, *e.g.*, / a ... or multiple occurrences of a member of Group A, "the / the / the ..." with no noun following. All this amounts to further support for the observation that FP and UP are not functionally different since they both precede most often either a single noun or a noun phrase. Also the aphasics share with the normals in this patterned distribution (P-N; P-NP) which again brings into relief the non-qualitative difference of the aphasic disorder.

Goldman-Eisler (1964) commented that "Pausing might thus be the behaviour concomitant of processes in the brain concerned with verbal planning and selection," (p. 99) proposing that hesitation pauses divide speech into cognitive categories. (p. 103) There is hardly any empirical foundation, at the present time at least, for such a broad generalization. This claim is also not amenable to direct testing.

On the other hand, the results provide data on the problem of what constitutes the fundamental functioning unit of encoding in speech production. Both in psychology and linguistics this crucial process is not yet fully understood. Encoding in a non-afflicted speaker seems to be an ongoing coordination of vocal-verbal sequences that are performed so fluently in time that the listener is almost unaware of the complexity of the final output. Yet there will always be points where the speaker self-interrupts the linguistic stream, where decisions about what to say next are being made internally.

In the light of the findings of this study, considerable evidence supports the position that the noun phrase, consisting of the two constituents D and N, functions as this psycholinguistic unit of encoding. This observation is strictly derived from overt speech behavior. Non-speech periods in spontaneous speech characteristically occur where the following verbal sequence involves a member of the class of determiners plus a lexical item of Class 1. This view is further reinforced by the fact that at least 50% of the members of Class 1 were subject personal pronouns which are often abbreviated realizations of noun phrases. A study by Brown and Bellugi (1964) touches upon this very fact in their discussion of the evolution of the Noun Phrase in child speech. They write "The words called 'pronouns' in English would more aptly be called 'pro-noun-phrases' since it is the phrase rather than the noun which they usually replace." (p. 150) Moreover, they found that children's pause occurrences usually enclose the NP as a self-contained unit.[1] Osgood and Maclay (1959) provide additional support in this direction when reporting results on another hesitation variable, false start. These experimenters point out that "When False Starts are retraced, it is usually a lexical item that is corrected, but the speaker also includes the closely associated function words in his retracing. This would suggest that at some level of organization the encoding unit is phrase-like, a lexical core with its tightly bound grammatical context." (p. 40-41)

We argue only that the NP is one of the determining units underlying the encoding process in spontaneous speech production and that pauses might be viewed as significant concomitant markers to identify this unit. One can say, at least for English, that hesitation pauses are complementary determinants in a speaker's linguistic performance for this typical configuration of syntax, the noun phrase.

Thus it has been demonstrated by this research that the aphasic dysfunction does not break down this basic encoding unit of noun or noun phrase preceded by either FP or UP. These structural properties are, rather, preserved.

[1] Most recent attempts to account for syntactic structures in linguistic theory through the categories of symbolic logic has led George Lakoff to a position that would eliminate VP as a syntactic category from the structural descriptions of sentences. If this step can be taken at all, it would leave NP as the ultimate linguistic unit.

APPENDIX 1

TWO SAMPLE TRANSCRIPTS OF APHASIC SPEECH

Aphasic Patient A4

He's [ə] hollerin', / he has a cap / and a jacket / and he's / he's [ə] / oh, livin' on the fence. / He's got [ə] / pants on / and she he's got something o-on the shirt / and he a-hangin' on / the rail / or the /fence.

On number 2, / they's a lady and a man. / He's he's got a hat on / and the 'nother man is [ə] / 's got a / f-he is holding something in here hands / and the lady's got a / the broom / and he's she's got a hat on.

Three, / she's got two boys / and [ə] / she got a, / she's got a / sweater on and [ə] the boy has [ə] / he's got a ch- a shirt on / and she's got [ə] kerchief on her hair. / The ba- the boy he's got curly hair. / That's all.

Number 4, / he's got a / bash cloth, / she's [ə] / cleanin' the boy's face, her ear / and [ə] / the dirl is got a / pribbon in here here her hair / and [ə] / and she has a dog / with a clowel over his hair [ə] head / and she's got [ə] / slippers / in her his her feet. / The wash cloth, / the soap / in the water.

Five, five, / it's [ə] / he's the the water the / [ə] the beach / and he's got his [ə] around / the girl. / She has a cap, the / and the d- the lady's got his / arm over the / on the the shoulder of the boy / and / she got [ə] / his shoes are all tied up / and / she's got a bracelet on her his [ə] her arm.

Aphasic Patient A5

One, / the boy he was / maybe he was [ə] / scream or something but he was [ə] just sitting. / I guess the somebody was playing but he [ə] / it was warm / but there is nothing too much. / Just a boy he was just [ə] / talk or scream something and they were playing and he said "Stop" or. / But it's [ə] really not too much.

Two. / Well there's a girl and I guess she was playing. / Her / this man he is [ə] / curtain, no, [ə]. / I guess this is a boy but I guess he wasn't playing but [ə] he is [ə] his face [ə] / he was going to a / movies or something just playing. / And the girl she has a old / dress. Maybe it was a mother or / grandma's. / He hair it's [ə] / a hat / [m̩] and I guess there's nothing then.

Three. / There was a / a lady. She has a mother and she has a b-two boys, / two boys? Oh, no, there's a boy and a girl / and [ə] / they're not [ə] / just tal- [ə] / standing. / But it's getting dark / and we don't know if it's a maybe school or something with old. / or not ol'. Something is old I guess.

This is girl and boy. The girl she was [ə] the boy / here is a she was cleanin' and [ə] there's a dog / and there's [ə] soap / and the girl has [ə] / cleanes the the boy / hearing. / I don't think the boy he was mad / but the girl she was helping.

Five. / There's two girls and a boy. / He's in the army / and then have one girls he was just a kiss. / Another girl she was [ə] just [ə] the water. / I guess it was warm. / I would say it's a bad Saturday but they don't have to work and s- and Sunday they have to don't church. So they're just [ə] / just sit and kiss and / OK.

APPENDIX 2

SAMPLE OF PAUSE LENGTHS PRINT-OUT FROM IBM 360 COMPUTER

A1			A2		
TIME	LENGTH	SYNC	TIME	LENGTH	SYNC
.06	.08		.09	.10	
1.08	.04		1.22	.14	
1.14	2.38		1.68	2.66	
4.03	.94		4.51	1.14	
5.71	5.20		5.73	.10	
11.19	1.54	1	6.11	.10	
12.78	.04		6.92	.16	
12.86	.16		7.10	11.30	
13.27	.04		18.57	.52	1
13.41	10.16		19.27	.26	
24.05	4.08	2	19.73	.06	
28.44	3.18		19.96	.12	
32.00	1.28	3	20.34	.06	2
33.61	1.60		20.71	.06	
35.71	12.90		20.79	.02	
48.97	1.50	4	21.09	1.12	
50.92	.56	5	22.42	.04	
51.66	1.22		22.80	.68	
53.49	12.28		23.67	.74	
65.95	1.40	6	25.33	1.28	
67.67	.12		26.85	.12	
68.12	.08		27.38	1.40	
68.56	.24		28.80	1.22	
68.93	.16		30.29	.18	3
69.51	2.44		30.69	.20	
72.23	5.42	7	31.09	.12	
78.00	.08		31.42	.06	
78.50	.08		31.50	1.02	
79.23	2.82		33.27	.94	
82.39	8.54	8	34.61	.20	
91.47	.96	9	35.33	.10	

92.60	.14		35.58	.16	
93.24	.04		36.04	.08	
93.57	5.86		36.53	.08	
99.67	2.96		36.77	.12	
103.17	1.62	10	37.39	.62	
105.00	5.78		38.10	.12	
111.28	.64	11	38.24	.04	
112.51	.58		38.55	.52	
113.43	1.78		39.59	.52	
115.67	3.82		40.61	3.24	4
120.08	.08	12	44.28	.04	
120.72	.36		44.34	.22	
121.13	.66		44.59	.08	
121.93	.80		45.01	.10	
123.25	.60		45.69	.86	
124.22	.74		46.60	7.12	
125.22	.28		53.98	.26	5
125.53	.92				
126.83	2.16				
129.61	.14				
129.80	.02				
130.16	5.08	13			
135.55	2.74				
138.53	.16				
138.97	1.26				
140.64	.94	14			
141.90	.30				
142.61	1.04				
144.01	.90				
145.17	2.20				
148.10	.02				
148.16	.03				

APPENDIX 3

SAMPLE OF FREQUENCY DISTRIBUTION OF PAUSE DURATIONS

Normal Control Subject N5

PROGRAM RESTART

AVE =	.97416497		SD = 1.3866821			MODE = .32000000			MEDIAN = .88000000		
NUM =	535		SUM = 579.15999			LONGP =	0		KSHORT =	2564	
.26	21	.28	19	.30	17	.32	21	.34	8	.36	12
.38	8	.40	12	.42	8	.44	7	.46	16	.48	14
.50	9	.52	3	.54	6	.56	9	.58	4	.60	3
.62	4	.64	4	.66	7	.68	6	.70	8	.72	4
.74	4	.76	7	.78	6	.80	4	.82	6	.84	5
.86	4	.88	8	.90	7	.92	9	.94	3	.96	5
.98	4	1.00	5	1.02	5	1.04	7	1.06	4	1.08	7
1.10	3	1.12	4	1.14	6	1.16	4	1.18	1	1.20	3
1.22	7	1.24	4	1.26	6	1.28	3	1.30	6	1.32	3
1.34	4	1.36	2	1.38	8	1.40	5	1.42	5	1.44	5
1.46	3	1.48	1	1.50	1	1.52	6	1.54	8	1.56	7
1.58	2	1.60	1	1.62	1	1.64	6	1.66	2	1.68	1
1.70	2	1.72	2	1.74	2	1.76	3	1.78	1	1.80	2
1.82	4	1.84	1	1.86	2	1.88	2	1.90	1	1.96	5
2.00	2	2.02	1	2.04	1	2.08	2	2.10	4	2.16	1
2.18	1	2.20	1	2.24	2	2.28	1	2.32	1	2.36	1
2.38	2	2.40	1	2.42	1	2.48	2	2.50	1	2.52	1
2.54	1	2.66	1	2.68	1	2.70	1	2.72	1	2.74	1
2.78	1	2.90	1	2.94	1	3.00	1	3.02	2	3.04	2
3.06	1	3.24	1	3.30	2	3.34	1	3.38	1	3.40	1
3.44	1	3.46	1	3.50	1	3.54	1	3.62	1	3.80	1
4.10	1	4.38	1	4.74	1	4.92	1	5.60	1	6.00	1
6.02	1										

END OF JOB

SAMPLE OF OSCILLOGRAPH RECORD

Aphasic Patient A6

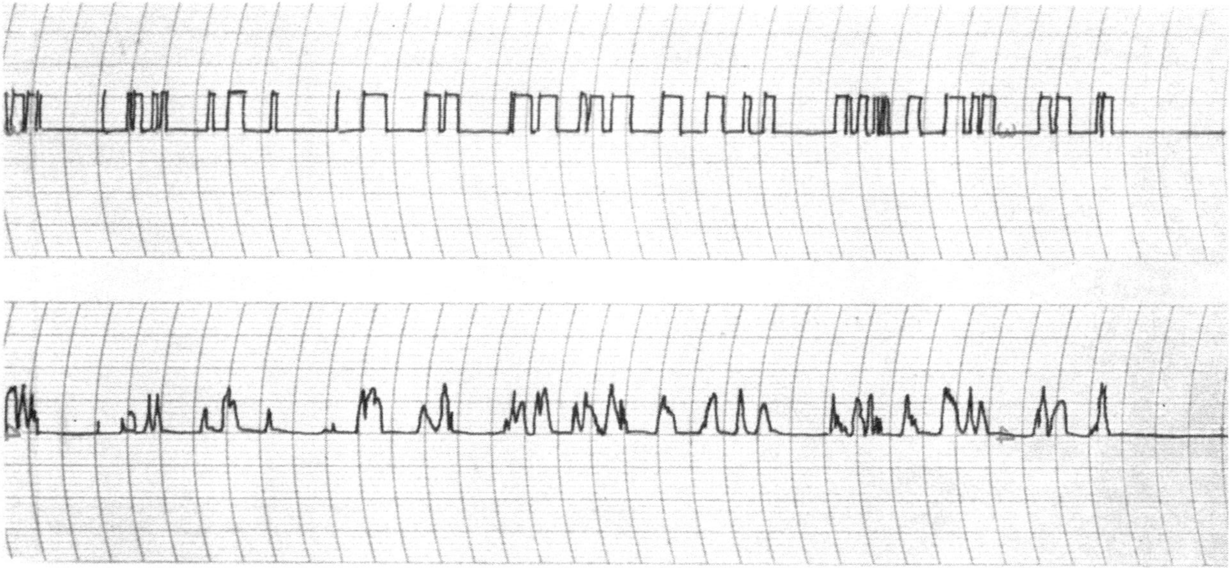

Upper pen tracing indicates digital data
Lower pen tracing indicates relative speech data displaying amplitudes
Temporal scale: 1 box equals 1 second

REFERENCES

Birdwhistell, Ray L.

1965 "Communication: a continuous multi-channel process", Draft: Chapter for *Conceptual Bases and Applications of the Communicationa Sciences*. University of California: Mimeographed (quoted with permission of author).

Blankenship, Jane and Kay, Christian

1964 "Hesitation phenomena in English speech: a study in distribution", *Word* 20, 360-372.

Bloomfield, Leonard

1933 *Language* (New York: Holt, Rinehart and Winston).

Boomer, Donald S.

1965 "Hesitation and grammatical encoding", *Language and Speech* 8, 148-158.

Brady, Paul T.

1965 "A technique for investigating on-off patterns of speech", *Bell System Technical Journal* 44, 1-22.

Brown, Roger, and Bellugi, U.

1964 "Three processes in the child's acquisition of syntax", *Harvard Educational Review* 34, 133-151.

Carson, Daniel H., Carson, Florence E., and Tikofsky, Ronald S.

1968 "On learning characteristics of the adult aphasic", *Cortex* 4, 92-112.

Chomsky, Noam

1957 *Syntactic Structures* (The Hague: Mouton)

1965 *Aspects of the Theory of Syntax* (Cambridge: M.I.T. Press).

Chomsky, Noam, Halle, M., and Lukoff, Fred

1956 "On accent and juncture in English", *in*: Halle, M., and Lunt, H., and Mac Lean, H. (eds.), *For Roman Jakobson* (The Hague: Mouton), 65-80.

Chomsky, Noam, and Halle, Morris

1968 *The Sound Pattern of English* (New York: Harper & Row).

The Family of Man. 1955 (New York: Maco-Magazine Corporation).

Fries, C. C.

1952 *The Structure of English* (New York: Harcourt, Brace and World).

Gleason, H. A., Jr.
1961 *An Introduction to Descriptive Linguistics*, rev. ed. (New York: Holt, Rinehart and Winston).
Goldman-Eisler, F.
1955 "Speech-breathing activity—a measure of tension and affect during interviews", *British Journal of Psychology* 46, 53-63.
1958a "Speech analysis and mental processes", *Language and Speech* 1, 59-75.
1958b "Speech production and the predictability of words in context", *Quarterly Journal of Experimental Psychology* 10, 96-106.
1958c "The predictability of words in context and the length of pauses in speech", *Language and Speech* 1, 226-231.
1961a "A comparative study of two hesitation phenomena", *Language and Speech* 4, 18-26.
1961b "Hesitation and information in speech", in: Cherry, C. (ed.), *Information Theory—Fourth London Symposium* (London: Butterworth and Co.), 162-173.
1964 "Hesitation, information, and levels of speech production", in: de Reuck, A. V. S. and O'Connor, Maeve (eds.), *Ciba Foundation Symposium on Disorders of Language* (Boston: Little, Brown and Co.), 96-111.
Goodglass, H.
1962 "Redefining the concept of agrammatism in aphasia", in Croatto, L. and Croatto-Martinollí, C. (eds.), *Proceedings of the XIIth International Speech and Voice Therapy Conference* (Padua: Istituto Superiore Sordomuti E.N.S. A. Magarotto), 108-115.
Goodglass, H., and Hunt, J.
1958 "Grammatical complexity and aphasic speech", *Word* 14, 197-207.
Goodglass, H., and Berko Jean
1960 "Agrammatism and inflectional morphology in English", *Journal of Speech and Hearing Research* 3, 257-267.
Greenberg, Joseph H.
1965 "The word as a linguistic unit", in: Osgood, Charles E. and Sebeok, Thomas A. (eds.), *Psycholinguistics—A Survey of Theory and Research Problems* (Bloomington: Indiana University Press), 66-71.
Grewel, F.
1963 "Prolegomena to patholinguistics", in Halpern, Lipman (ed.), *Problems of Dynamic Neurology* (Jerusalem: Jerusalem Post Press), 71-87.
Hargreaves, William A. and Starkweather, John A.
1959 "Collection of temporal data with the duration tabulator", *Journal of the Experimental Analysis of Behavior* 2, 179-183.
Henderson, A., Goldman-Eisler, F., and Skarbek, Andrew
1966 "Sequential temporal patterns in spontaneous speech", *Language and Speech* 9, 207-216.
Hjelmslev, Louis
1927 *Principes de grammaire générale* (Copenhagen: Munksgaard).

1953 *Prolegomena to a Theory of Language*. Translated from the Danish, 1943, by Francis J. Whitfield (Bloomington: Indiana University Press).

Howes, Davis H.

1964 "Application of the word-frequency concept to aphasia", in: de Reuck, A. V. S. and O'Connor, Maeve (eds.), *Ciba Foundation Symposium on Disorders of Language* (Boston: Little, Brown and Co.), 47-75.

Jakobson, R.

1941 *Kindersprache, Aphasie und allgemeine Lautgesetze* (Uppsala: Almquist and Wiksells Boktryckeri A.-B.)

1955 "Aphasia as a linguistic problem", in Werner, H. (ed.), *On Expressive Language* (Worcester: Clark University Press), 69-81.

1964 "Towards a linguistic typology of aphasic impairments", in: de Reuck, A. V. S. and O'Connor, Maeve (eds.), *Ciba Foundation Symposium on Disorders of Language* (Boston: Little, Brown and Co.), 21-42.

Jakobson, R., and Halle, Morris

1956 *Fundamentals of Language* (The Hague: Mouton).

Jones, Lyle V. and Wepman, Joseph M.

1965 "Language: a perspective from the study of aphasia", in: Rosenberg, S. (ed.), *Directions in Psycholinguistics* (New York: Macmillan Co.), 237-253.

Lehrer, A.

1968 "Competence, grammaticality and sentence complexity", *The Philosophical Forum* 1, 85-89.

Lenneberg, Eric H.

1960 Review of *Speech and Brain Mechanisms*, by Wilder Penfield and Lamar Roberts. *Language* 36, 97-112.

Levin, Harry and Silverman, Irene

1965 "Hesitation phenomena in children's speech", *Language and Speech* 8, 67-85.

Livant, William P.

1963 "Antagonistic functions of verbal pauses: filled and unfilled pauses in the solution of additions", *Language and Speech* 6, 1-4.

Maclay, H. and Osgood, C. E.

1959 "Hesitation phenomena in spontaneous English speech", *Word* 15, 19-44.

Mahl, George F.

1956 "Disturbances and silences in the patient's speech in psychotherapy", *Journal of Abnormal and Social Psychology* 53, 1-15.

Miller, George A.

1963 *Language and Communication* (New York: McGraw-Hill Paperback).

Moulton, William G.

1947 "Juncture in modern German", in Joos, M. (ed.), *Readings in Linguistics* (New York: American Council of Learned Societies), 208-215.

Osgood, Charles E. and Miron, Murray S.

1963 *Approaches to the Study of Aphasia* (Urbana: University of Illinois Press).

Sapon, Stanley M.
1957 *A Pictorial Linguistic Interview Manual* (Columbus: Ohio State University).
Schwartz, Joseph and Jaffe, Joseph
1968 "Markovian prediction of sequential temporal patterns in spontaneous speech", *Language and Speech* 11, 27-30.
Smith, J. O. and Dunn, Lloyd
1965 *The Peabody Language Development Kit* (Minneapolis: American Guidance Service).
Tannenbaum, Percy H., Williams, F., and Hillier, Carolyn S.
1965 "Word predictability in the environments of hesitations", *Journal of Verbal Learning and Verbal Behavior* 4, 134-140.
Tannenbaum, Percy H., Williams, F., and Wood, Barbara S.
1967 "Hesitation phenomena and related encoding characteristics in speech and typewriting", *Language and Speech* 10, 203-215.
Tikofsky, R. S.
1966 "Language problems in adults", in Rieber, R. W. and Brubaker, R. S. (eds.), *Speech Pathology: An International Study of the Science* (Amsterdam: North-Holland Publishing Co.), 261-284.
Trager, G. L. and Smith, Henry Lee
1957 *An Outline of English Structure* (= *Studies in Linguistics, Occasional Papers*, No. 3.) (Washington, D.C.: American Council of Learned Societies).
Twaddell, W. F.
1959 "Linguistics plus", *Report of the Tenth Annual Round Table Meeting on Linguistics and Language Studies*, No. 12 (Washington, D.C.), 147-156.
Wepman, J. M., Bock, R. D., Jones, L. V., and Van Pelt, D.
1956 "Psycholinguistic study of aphasia: a revision of the concept of anomia", *Journal of Speech and Hearing Disorders* 21, 468-477.
Zipf, G. K.
1965 *The Psycho-biology of Language: An Introduction to Dynamic Philology* (Cambridge: First M.I.T. Press Paperback Edition).

INDEX

Bei Fragen zur Produktsicherheit wenden Sie sich bitte an:
If you have any questions regarding product safety,
please contact:

Walter de Gruyter GmbH
Genthiner Straße 13
10785 Berlin
productsafety@degruyterbrill.com